THE NEST OF SANITY

Rebecca Morgan

Rebecca Morgan

Published by
Chipmunkapublishing
PO Box 6872
Brentwood
Essex CM13 1ZT
United Kingdom

http://www.chipmunkapublishing.com

Copyright © Rebecca Morgan 2008

Cover illustration by Sue Shaw

Edited by Mary Dow

Chipmunkapublishing gratefully acknowledges the support of Arts Council England.

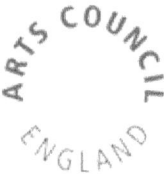

THE NEST OF SANITY

ACKNOWLEDGEMENTS

I wish to thank my brothers and my sister for their love, care and support through very difficult times. Thank you to my son for letting me tell a small part of his story.
I am indebted to my husband for his love, patience and understanding.
Similarly thank you to my good friends (you know who you are) for their love, support and listening skills. Thanks particularly to the coffee morning crowd for their support and encouragement.
Thanks also to the Off the Shelf Reading and Writing Festival in Sheffield which inspired me in 2007 to revisit my manuscript.
Finally thanks to Jason Pegler my publisher for his help and advice.

Rebecca Morgan

THE NEST OF SANITY

AUTHORS NOTE

Most of the names in this story have been changed to protect the privacy of family and friends. I do not intend to cause offence to any person by the writing of this book.

Rebecca Morgan

THE NEST OF SANITY

PREFACE

I have come to regard sanity as a nest. Within are the baby bird fledglings; safe, warm, cosy and comforted, fed and protected by their parents. But danger is real and ever present and it is only a short distance away. I myself have fallen from this nest four times in a space of twenty seven years, and I may well fall again. In this book I have tried to accurately recall my experiences during these episodes of madness in the hope that this will both enlighten those who are strangers to such illness and to comfort those fellow sufferers with the knowledge that they do not suffer alone. Finally I wish to offer inspiration in the form of hope that you can get better and lead a fulfilling and happy life.

Rebecca Morgan

THE NEST OF SANITY

This book is dedicated to Phyll and Taffy

Rebecca Morgan

THE NEST OF SANITY

CONTENTS

Rebecca Morgan

THE NEST OF SANITY

PART ONE

1980: SHEFFIELD

The taxi dropped me in front of the stone-fronted terraced houses. I walked up the five steps, along the brick passage and to the door. Tentatively, I put the key in the lock and turned it. There was a fresh smell to the hall, not like the musty aroma which usually hits you after leaving the house empty awhile. No doubt my mother had been cleaning. A gurgled murmur from the sling around my neck reminded me that the baby's feed was about due. For the first time I was home with my baby boy for good. Not quite a new-born baby, for he was over four months old.

As I unlaced the baby-sling and placed Steven carefully in his bouncing cradle, I marvelled at what a lovely baby he was. Contented and smiling even though he was hungry. I began to prepare the bottle, looking back over the first few months of Steven's life.

I could remember certain things, but much that had happened was just blankness in my mind. For I had spent three months in Middlewood, the local Psychiatric hospital and the Electro Convulsive Therapy* (ECT) had caused a period of amnesia – a sort of blanking out of the worst experiences. This failure of my memory was a weird and disturbing feature of the illness – at times I would panic if I could not recall an incident, face, name, any little thing. Frightening!   But I knew from experience that the memories would eventually revive and invade my mind in patchy outbursts. Suddenly, in the midst of normal everyday sequential thoughts, I would picture myself, say, hysterical, being calmed by a nurse after having ripped down the curtains of the hospital room. I would stop stock still, amazed, unbelieving that the incident had been real; then I would feel shock and horror and perhaps a hint of shame and I would store that fractional memory away with the rest: eating the yellow head of a daffodil; running away into the snowy street wearing only a nightdress; smashing a full dish of muesli and milk against my bedroom wall; sitting with my arms clasped around my knees, head bent, rocking back and forward humming to myself; believing I was communicating with my dead father by tapping on the hospital walls and fingering hot radiators. I knew the memories would return as they had before. For, the breakdown following my baby's birth was preceded by two others from which I made a full recovery.

(*Electro Convulsive Therapy is a controversial Psychiatric treatment in which seizures are induced with electricity for therapeutic effect. ECT is most often used as a treatment for severe major depression which has not responded to other treatment and is also used for treatment for schizophrenia and other related disorders.)

THE NEST OF SANITY

Steven's birth I could remember fairly well. I awoke at 3.30 a.m. on the very day the baby was due in January, 1980. I had diarrhoea and had to run to the toilet. I continued to go for about forty minutes, back and forth, and finally realised with some panic that the periodic cramp-like pains in my lower abdomen were labour pains.

After much effort I woke Ralph, my husband, and we packed a bag and got organised. The contractions were then coming every two to three minutes. The ambulance got us to the maternity hospital by about six o'clock and only one and a half hours later Steven was born. I suffered much pain, but was greatly helped by the breathing exercises and song-reciting which natural childbirth classes had taught me. I only once completely lost control when being told not to push whilst having an overbearing urge to do so.

After some worry that forceps might be needed to ease the baby's head out, a small episiotomy was done, I was able to push with tremendous effort and Steven was born screaming loudly. Ralph held my hand, comforted, encouraged and supported throughout. We were deliriously happy and excited and I wanted immediately to impart the news to all our close relatives, so Ralph rushed off with two pence pieces and phone numbers.

Immediately after the delivery, I felt very tired but elated. Indeed, at some points through the labour I had imagined I was above the bed watching down on myself. This may have been the effect of too much gas and air or perhaps a sign of things to come. The baby was healthy and weighed six pounds. He fitted exactly in the palms of Ralph's two hands. Steven, as we had decided to call him, wanted nothing but to sleep for twenty-four hours and I wonder, if I could have done the same, perhaps I would have fared better. My blood pressure was high and consequently I was not taken up to a ward for a few hours. I found the wards extremely hot which prevented me from sleeping. (It was 100 degrees Fahrenheit on the wall thermometer). My appetite was poor and little worries about the care of such a small human being all resulted in outbursts of tears. The nurses assured me this was natural: 'We all have the baby blues at first, dear'. I struggled on with feeds and nappy changes. I became extremely sore as baby Steven did not show any interest in feeding, but was regularly woken from his postnatal slumbers and 'hooked' onto my tender breasts. The nights were gruelling, with four babies in each bay taking turns at screaming. I got little chance to rest, and anyway, I was so uncomfortably hot and so mentally on edge that I could not go to sleep.

After two or three days, I was moved to a side ward of my own. I was becoming increasingly confused and unrelated to the reality of the situation. I was desperate to return home and kept making endless nonsensical lists of what I needed urgently to do. I refused to see any visitors except my husband, and I broke down every time he had to leave me. I felt that I was beginning some sort of breakdown, but the nursing staff had little time or patience with my concerns. One doctor, however, who had stitched me up after the episiotomy, listened to my considerable and involved worries for some hours one evening. Next day I wrote him a thank you note, as I felt he alone had saved me from a downward slide into illness.

After the usual seven day stay in the maternity hospital, I remember coming home in a taxi with Ralph and my mother, but I did not at that point really understand even that I had had a baby, let alone that I should care for it. I denied any recollection of the labour and birth and disowned Steven. I refused to feed him and preferred not to have too much to do with him. My Mum, who came to stay for a few days, ended up staying for four months. Together with Ralph, she took on the role of surrogate mother, bottle feeding and nappy changing, during the hectic comings and goings of midwives, health visitors, doctors, friends, neighbours and well wishers, while my condition further deteriorated.

I was behaving uncharacteristically and, although a non-smoker, smoked a whole packet of

Park Drive begged from a neighbour. I was
restless and over excited.

In the midst of all this, I received two pieces
of news which deeply distressed me. A close
friend, who was expecting a baby in March that
year, had a stillborn little girl a few days after
Steven's birth. Two years previously she had
given birth to a baby boy who only lived for two
days. Then, a friend of mine called Steve, who
lived in South Devon sent me a birthday card
which disclosed that he had been diagnosed as
having Multiple Sclerosis. I responded to this by
actually starting to chew the birthday card in the
misguided hope that I could 'eat his words',
thereby rendering them untrue.

During this time, I would not wash or look
after myself. I did not want to eat but swallowed
endless cups of sugary tea.   I have been told that
at one point I talked continuously for four days and
nights, and I could not be persuaded to try to
sleep. My brother-in-law sat with me for twenty
four hours and I responded to his cajoling by
tipping a jug of cold water over his head. I was
relieved to see my reliable GP and let him into the
house while I was totally naked. I told him I loved
him and threw my bare arms around him.   He
called a Psychiatrist, who apparently saw me,
again nude, cleaning out the bathroom cupboard.
This chore took me three hours of sorting, moving
and adjusting the contents in an endless search

for the ideal arrangement. I could not be persuaded to stop.

I remember believing that I was being taken to a Mother and Baby club as I was driven away with a social worker and a doctor on a dismal rainy night to the local mental hospital, Middlewood. I could not comprehend that I had been Sectioned. (Sectioning is a very scary process but I was oblivious to what was happening.) This hospital was universally feared in Sheffield, but I have to say everyone was marvellous to me there. After a week in a single room, I was joined by baby Steven and placed in a three bed unit specifically for postnatal mums with three cots, three prams and all facilities for the care of babies. I didn't realise till later that it was beneficial to share with women in a similar situation, for together we were able to help each other with the tricky business of coping with new born children. The staff were very caring and supportive and all became very fond of Steven. They often left me to sleep at night, while they dealt with nappy changing and feeds. I shared the unit with an Asian Mum, Shamim, who later had a second baby and a second postnatal breakdown.

On the larger ward there were patients with a range of problems. I do remember one or two quite clearly. I made friends with Edith, who suffered from agoraphobia. She would tremble with panic in open spaces and when I felt better, I used to help her run blindly across to the

Occupational Therapy building, only a few yards away. Margery, a lady in her thirties, seemed quite an ordinary woman until you noticed her arms. She spent much of her waking day stubbing lighted cigarettes out on the skin of her wrists. Careful rows of burns, little round burns, lined up on her arms. To see her do this was awful, but she seemed to suffer the pain with an excitement which made it all worth doing. I once came across her slashing her wrists in the shower. I was horrified by the sight of so much blood and rushed to the nurses' station, blurting out what had happened. Margery left the hospital a few weeks before I did and I thought that was the last I would see of her, but the day before I was to be discharged, she was back, burn marks and all, as bad as before.

During those weeks I was not at first in touch with reality. I suffered from delusions such as believing I was the daughter of Jesus and spent some time in the old church in the grounds of the hospital. The minister was very patient and kind to me. It was only the ECT which erased those delusions. Also I was treated with the drug largactyl, which I took as a medicine as I had refused to take injections. I was very frightened of needles, which had resulted in violent struggles during which I resisted the treatment.

I was to stay at Middlewood Hospital as an in-patient for four months. I soon took part in occupational activities like rug-making, knitting and poetry writing. I also used to play table tennis particularly with my brother-in-law who loved competitive sport. I believed that all the patients and nurses were controlled by a higher being and that we were all suffering the after effects of a nuclear war. I used to read aloud from an old Bible in the patient's lounge, which must have been annoying to others. I often blocked the showers with tissue paper and poured full bottles of shampoo down the plug holes. It was all part of a plan I felt I had to follow to appease the Gods. Man had spoilt nature with pollution: I had to cleanse the world.

My mother, husband and friends visited regularly. My best friend Anne and Jane, my librarian friend, came every week. Gradually, over many weeks and by having ECT I emerged from the worst of my psychosis, and with pills and therapy I was able to recover slowly and to learn how to love my son and how to cope with the daily routine of caring for him. No-one had warned me about the possibility of postnatal problems though I had heard of the baby blues. I had thought that a mum would automatically love her child but in my case it wasn't true. I had to work on those feelings and eventually felt great warmth and love for my son.

When I finally left the hospital, I was helped marvellously by Health Visitors and Community Liaison staff. I found though that I totally lacked self confidence and did not really want to leave the house. My Health Visitor came every day at first , helped me with feeding and bathing Steven and gave me one of the most useful tips for leading an active and depression free life. She advised me to make a daily list of chores/visits/outings. Ticking off even a small chore made me feel more purposeful and satisfied; and she advised me to plan the week ahead making sure I had something to look forward to each day, even if only a visit to the local Clinic. This may seem very basic and obvious, but I was struggling and not coping very well and I was perpetually tired.

In those first few weeks at home I felt strange, lonely and tearful, but slowly I became a bit more adventurous and broached local Mother and Baby and then Mother and Toddler Groups. There, gradually, I found renewed confidence once I had made friends amongst mothers, who had sometimes also suffered from Post Natal Depression. (Many of these are still friends today.)

During the first few months, I had moments when I felt inadequate, lost and un-loving towards my husband and my baby. I will admit I even shook Steven once or twice, but never actually harmed him. (I can sympathise with postnatal mothers who lose control.) I had the support and help of neighbours and friends and the unceasing love and care of my husband, who was coping with night shifts at a local factory where he was a machinist. My mother showed her true and loyal colours by staying for four months until she felt I could cope. I could not have managed without her.

A lot of that period of my life is a blur in my memory, but it still remains a traumatic time. I had had a postnatal Psychotic breakdown (called Puerperal Psychosis by the doctors.) I was advised by my Psychiatrist to continue my medication for the rest of my life and also not to have another child as the probability was that, with my medical history, I would have another breakdown.

PART TWO

1971: SHEFFIELD

Looking back, I feel that I had been building up to a breakdown for several years, perhaps even as far back as my early childhood. I was born in Hoddesdon in Hertfordshire in 1951 and came from a big family. I had three brothers and a sister so there were seven of us altogether, plus various pets along the way. I was the middle one amongst the five children and the most sensitive. They were happy times but sometimes stressful due to the lack of money in the household. Perhaps I was sensitive because of my father's strict regime.

I remember my father with love and fondness, I remember my baby brother sitting gurgling on his knee while he chuckled him under the chin. But I remember too his tempers, his strictness and his drinking. He was born in the valleys of South Wales and spent his early years working down the coalmines. He ran away to London when he was twenty and started sweeping up on the hairdresser's floor. After some time he had his own barber's shop. On his afternoons off, he drank at home and the alcohol used to bring on various moods, anger, hot temper and morose depression, in sequence. When his temper cooled he used to dwell on his childhood, his family of nine children, two of whom died in

THE NEST OF SANITY

childhood. In adult life two of his sisters died of cancer. He was the sort of man who would do his mates any favour, loan money, let them bed down for the night. He was a socialist in his views and a convinced atheist. He worked very hard for his family and was devoted to my mother. He tried to give us good advice for our future lives. Yet he was very strict and we feared his homecomings. He would take off his thick leather belt and chase us, lashing out if we had been naughty. Usually we were too nimble and escaped, hiding under the table or behind the door. We used to play up to my Mum, but a cry of 'Dad's coming!' would stop the pranks while we hurriedly straightened the table where we had been improvising a game of table tennis or the cushions and chairs of our den.

My Mum was born in a village in Essex. She was of a nervous disposition and didn't have much confidence. She was usually tired and harassed with five children close in age. She was on the go from morning to night. It was only in later years that my mum learned to relax, grew in confidence and came into her own. She was a loving and caring mother to all her children.

I was often moody and grizzly as a child, prone to outbursts of temper if I wanted my own way. I used to get very worked up and sometimes banged my head against the wall. I was bright at school, but found it hard to make friends. Often my playmates were much younger than me. As a child, I was shy and quiet and spent much time lost in a book. Once I learnt to read, I devoured books and visited the library every week.

I was conscientious with my school work to the extent that I would worry considerably about it and often could not sleep. I suffered from insomnia regularly and often missed school to catch up on sleep. The crunch came at age fifteen, when the doctor prescribed sleeping pills because I could not rest with the O Level exams on my mind. I literally used to toss and turn all night and felt exhausted in the mornings. The GP also wanted to prescribe some tranquilisers to calm me down but I was alarmed and worried that they were addictive. (Perhaps if I had taken those pills then, I may have been spared mental health problems later in life?) At eighteen I left home for Sheffield University, and was very homesick. I could not afford to visit home very often and at first had trouble making friends. I had led a very sheltered life and did not have the confidence for all the new social situations which arose. I found the kind of life and the self-disciplined approach quite strange and hard-going. I did settle in however, made friends and participated actively in the social and academic life that opened up for me. I took up new hobbies, joined a tenpin bowling team, became secretary of the film club, enjoyed dancing and had a few boyfriends. Then I fell in love for the first time and was concerned by the conflicts this caused in me. Trevor was a student three years older than me, a Yorkshire lad, charming but stubborn and moody. Lazy, but witty and clever. I was to date him for six years, but his uneven temperament and his unreliability did not bring out the best in me. However, for the meantime, I thought he was marvellous.

During the second year of the course, when I became ill, I had no examinations and therefore, there was no added pressure. I did have emotional problems with my first serious boyfriend, Trevor, and I feel that was a contributory factor, but a major cause may have been the separation from my family.

I remember becoming more and more depressed over the early months of that year, 1971, when I was twenty. My boyfriend, who lived away from Sheffield, used to come for weekends, but I found the leave-taking unbearable. I used to cry and plead with him not to go. During the day, I would find myself bursting into tears for no apparent reason; if asked why I was crying, I would have no answer. I took to spending more time alone in my small attic bed sitter. I began to lag behind with essays and other set work.

The student health doctor listened carefully and prescribed tranquilisers, telling me not to work too hard, and not to worry. My general health deteriorated and I was living on junk food and not looking after myself properly. In June I developed tonsillitis, with an aching head and limbs, feeling hot and cold. The same doctor prescribed anti-biotics and recommended a couple of days' rest, suspecting it was glandular fever. I retired to my bed, with one or two friends waiting on me with cups of tea and meals, though my appetite was poor.

That Friday night there was to be a student ball, a big annual event at Trevor's old Hall of Residence, Crewe Hall. The doctor said I could attend provided I kept off all alcohol and did not overdo things. I sat up into the early hours sewing a long dress to befit the occasion.

The music was deafening. Countless bobbing figures jigged up and down to the strains of The Troggs. I hesitated at the edge of the dance floor. I had spent nearly a week in bed, going from hot and clammy to freezing cold. My throat was sore and my neck glands ached and throbbed. I had made a supreme effort to get to the ball. Now, somebody asked me to dance. I felt more like collapsing than dancing but took a deep breath, stepped forward and joined the heaving throng of sweating bodies. I started to jig my body from side to side, waving my arms to the disco beat. Suddenly the strobes started: green, red, blue, yellow. As the lights flashed and changed, my vision became clouded as people's movements distorted into short punctuated jerks around me. My head was spinning and something seemed to crack inside my brain. My mouth was open and a girl was screaming close by; so close I turned, but there was no-one, no-one… I had to get out; I must try to escape. The colours flashed before my eyes and I saw the ceiling, walls and floor revolve before me so that I could no longer tell which was which. I had collapsed. I was carried to a student room nearby and laid on the bed. The screaming was still ringing in my ears, but the room was deathly silent. Trevor and a friend stood over me in hushed concern. Someone proffered a glass of water.

We spent that night with some friends at Fulwood. I lay in bed shivering and sweating with my teeth constantly chattering. I felt completely terrified, but did not know why. I begged Trevor to stay with me, not to leave me for a moment. I kept saying how scared I was, but could not explain the feeling.

Early the next morning, the Student Health doctor was called. He seemed confused, concerned and almost angry that I had stayed the night away from my own flat. He took more interest in that fact than in how I felt. He muttered that perhaps I should not have gone to a ball if I had been feeling so off colour. He could not find anything physically wrong, but could see I was overwrought, so recommended that I be admitted to Ranmoor Clinic, a sick bay attached to one of the more modern student halls.

I remember vividly leaving our friends' house and the hem of my maroon maxi coat knocking over two pints of milk which smashed all over the step. I was so upset by this trivial

incident that I could not stop crying. I felt
desperately sad and in my diary I wrote "I am sunk
into depths of grief".

THE NEST OF SANITY

DARKNESS

I am lost in blinding darkness
Sometimes.
Pain-filled fearful moments
Crowd my very being.
A panic, sudden, bleak,
Terrorizes my body.
It passes…

Swept with heave of sorrow
The endless, endless tears
Rack at my heart.
Sorrow aggravating sorrow;
The overflowing emptiness
Of solitude.

Why can't you help me?
Why can't they see?
Life is strangely coloured
With dim reality.

Desperation follows, helplessly
Fighting always fighting
To conquer depths unknown.
Dimly light rejoins me,
Helplessness falls cautiously
Aside.
Emotion all but spent,
Drained relief – but oh
The fear of darkness's rebirth.

1971, Churchill Clinic, Harlow

Rebecca Morgan

I spent a week in Ranmoor Clinic, where I felt terribly isolated and low in spirits. I had several visitors, but I found the nursing staff rather short with me and not very understanding when I burst into tears several times a day. Close friends listened carefully as I ranted on about inconsequential things. The Doctor who came to see me said he could find nothing wrong with me at all. Later that evening I became hysterical and spent a restless night of panic and terror.

I passed a couple of days at my flat, after being discharged from the sick bay. I rested in bed, not eating, trying not to think, in an effort to clear my mind of confused jumble. Trevor managed to come and stay for the weekend, but, when Sunday evening came and he had to return to Coventry, I went berserk, screaming and tearing at his clothes. A doctor was called and he gave me an injection. A few moments later, on being helped to the toilet, I passed out on the floor. I vividly remember the awful giddiness before I fainted. Trevor afterwards said I went as yellow as the bathroom wallpaper.

The next day, with Trevor gone, I was inconsolable. A close friend came to take me out for a ride to the countryside, but I became hysterical in the confines of his sports car and the outing was disastrous. Also at this time, I had a strong fear of dogs, to the point of being panicky if

32

THE NEST OF SANITY

I saw one in the distance. Despite support from friends, I felt that I needed my family and struggled out to a call-box to telephone my sister Caroline in Manchester. She, not knowing of anything that had passed, refused to come immediately to see me and told me that I would be all right. (In retrospect she obviously did not realise the state I was in as I had concealed my problems from my family.) Finally, I rang a good friend, Lesley, at her home in Hertfordshire and she dropped everything and travelled up to Sheffield the next day to help. As it was almost vacation time, we decided Lesley would help me travel home. My belongings were packed and with Lesley and a University friend, Alison, I managed the journey home to Hertfordshire on the train. I'm not sure how I stood that journey, for I was still claustrophobic and hated being confined in the carriage. Also, the crowds at St. Pancras terrified me and I had to be physically supported, trembling, along the bustling platform.

Lesley's father met us there and drove us directly to my parents' house in Broxbourne, where I refused to see my father and insisted on being installed upstairs in my bedroom. (My illness and strange behaviour must have been a shock to my parents, from whom I had made every effort to conceal my depression of the past few months.) There, I spent several days, perhaps even weeks, eating little, sleeping, crying, and talking to my family, except my Dad, who had

suffered a serious stroke a few months previously
and whom I could not bear to face.

I saw my bedroom as a haven, an
impenetrable place of peace and calm. I got my
younger brother Graham to install a bell push so I
could summon help, food or company when ever I
needed it. No-one was allowed into my room
without knocking. I had by my bed the
tranquilisers prescribed for me, and I remember
taking them continuously, failing to regard the
dosage instructions. (This drug ingestion was
probably the cause of hallucinations, such as
feeling as though I was flying down hospital
corridors and seeing vivid patterns of colour spin
around my hospital room.) After some time, my
eldest brother Henry and my Mum persuaded me
to see a Psychiatrist. Throughout these
experiences, it must have been a great strain on
my family as they had never seen anyone in such
a state, while I was oblivious and in my own world.

THE NEST OF SANITY

1971: HARLOW

As my brother Henry drove me to the local hospital, I talked about subjects which normally would have embarrassed me, but which I felt I had to unburden onto someone. Mum sat in the front and flinched as I blurted out: "I have been on the pill for six months!" I had kept it a secret that I had been sleeping with my boyfriend as I knew my parents, particularly my Dad, would not approve. My Mum's face now looked concerned and anxious.

The hospital corridors were pale and dingy. We sat for a while in a waiting room and then I went in alone to see the Doctor. My idea of 'The Psychiatrist' loomed large in my mind – I had pictured him as middle-aged and serious, sitting behind a desk – and he was. Dr. T, as I shall call him, had greying hair thinly combed over his forehead. His eyes were warm and his expression kind. Before he could so much as say 'Hallo', I began:
"I know exactly what is wrong with me, and I have made notes to that effect":
I handed him a well-fingered page of file paper. I pointed out the salient lines –
"Symptom: Fear of dogs. Cause: Pet dog put to sleep when I was thirteen.
Symptom: Depression. Cause: Father's recent stroke, row with boyfriend etc"
Dr. T. smiled a wry smile, screwed up the piece of paper and dropped it in the waste bin.

"Well, I'm sure you meant to help, but really I just want to talk to you. Now then, you're a student, have you been having examinations this year?"

He questioned me generally, and then more specifically on my recent illness, academic record and social life. Then, he dismissed me, assuring me I would see him again soon, and asking me to send in my brother and mother. I sat in the waiting room somewhat perplexed. For a start, Dr. T. had taken little notice of the notes I had prepared for him. In fact, he had not even read them and now they were adding to the contents of his waste bin. Suddenly, I felt frightened, that cold panicky feeling which tightly grips you, leaving no room for breath. What could he be saying to Mum and Henry? What were they planning? He had mentioned a Clinic – Surely not a stay in Hospital?

On the drive home I was quiet. Mum briefly explained that Dr. T. had recommended a Psychiatric clinic in Harlow called The Churchill Clinic. He felt I would not improve without specialised care. What on earth would that entail I wondered? My mind boggled, and, finally, with the sway of the car, I fell asleep, curled up on the back seat in the now customary foetal position.

****

I lay back against the pillows as the melodies of familiar pop tunes washed over my clouded brain. I had shared this room with my

THE NEST OF SANITY

sister, Caroline, from an early age, and it was her tastes which still dominated its décor, even though she had left for Teacher Training College and a future in Cheshire four years before. Faded Elvis posters still hung on the cupboard door and her idol's name was engraved with pinpricks on the white painted window ledge at my side. I missed her and I missed my middle brother Stuart, who was currently travelling abroad with a friend.

The radio music stopped and the DJ introduced an item on Australia and a boy of twelve, who was fighting for his life with muscular dystrophy. Australia, that's where Stuart was working, selling lemonade, before trekking back on his route around the world. The boy's voice sent a panic through me – it was Stuart's voice, Stuart as he was when a boy. No, no, what did it mean? Stuart must have the disease and no-one had told me. He'd suffered thirteen years of illness and they had kept it from me. Oh, God, Stuart, please don't die – please come back and help me. With great force I threw the transistor radio to the floor, at first sobbing and then screaming in terror. No, help – it's Stuart - Oh God, he can't be dead – dead already, and they didn't tell me!! By the time my mother burst into the room, I was in complete hysteria and it was only a short sharp slap on the face which halted it.

The ambulance arrived shortly afterwards. Shaking, I clung to my mother's arm all the way to the hospital, pleading with her not to die. For she was Stuart and Stuart needed me; Stuart was dying.

At the Clinic the Psychiatrist took me into a side cubicle and tried to calm me down. He then left me with a nurse and escorted my mother to the office. Distraught, I called her back, but the nurse restrained me. The injection made me drowsy and I slept for a while. As I awoke, I heard clearly a woman's sobs from along the corridor. My mother, they were hurting my mother! Blindly, I half slipped, half fell off the bed and careered out of the room down the corridor. I burst into a small cubicle, shouting hysterically. A woman, a stranger, was crying near the door, comforted by a nurse. Two auxiliaries came up to me from behind and guided me, helpless, back to my room. They told me that my mother had left a while before and had long since returned home. I must 'calm down, for everything would be all right'.

My thoughts were in turmoil and I felt exhausted. I tried to keep hold of the truth behind the day's events. Stuart was ill, he may be dead. How much more was kept from me? What was I to do?

****

After being Sectioned, I spent about three months in the Clinic. It has all blurred in my memory as a time of long, dull days consisting of meals, meds and sleep. During the early days, I completely lost control of my bladder. I used to wet the floor; dull puddles into which other patients often wandered by mistake. The nurse would admonish me and order me off to the cupboard at the end of the corridor to fetch the mop and bucket. I remember one shameful night when I messed the bed and was thrown bodily into a hot bath the following morning. I felt very ashamed, but I was still confused as to what was really going on. I used to flush perfectly good panties down the hospital toilets; I lost lots of pairs that way.

Initially, I was largely confined to my room. I saw no other patients, only the nurses who came regularly to administer drugs and food. I was given sedatives and was encouraged to sleep, which I was grateful for. After a period of weeks, I began to feel a bit better and ventured from my room once or twice to the patients' lounge, where brightly coloured arm chairs were grouped around low coffee tables. Here, the patients watched television, listened to the radio, which was piped through two loud speakers, played cards and drank endless cups of tea. Most of the inmates were absent for a large part of the day. I later learned that they attended Occupational Therapy in another part of the building. The patients varied in age from a young girl of seventeen who had taken an overdose, to an old lady of eighty, confused and depressed after her husband, a vicar, had died. There was a woman (perhaps in her thirties and who had two small children) who was convinced that she had cancer, despite the tests which had proved negative. There were a couple of alcoholics trying to 'dry out' and a girl with the slimming disease anorexia nervosa.

At first I wanted no communication with the other inmates. I was preoccupied with my own form of unreality. I wasn't very interested in the problems of others, and only gradually over the weeks learned of their individual situations. One patient sticks in my memory. Jeremy must have been nearly forty years of age and yet he had shoulder length silver-grey hair and a silver ear-ring in one earlobe. Jeremy's problem was drugs - I was never quite sure what type of drugs, but I was told he was trying to 'kick the habit'. He spent much of his time in bed, with the covers pulled over his head. When he did emerge, he would regale us with stories of the time he worked with The Beatles. If you doubted his word, he used to fetch his tattered copy of the White Album, pull out the photo insert sheet and point to the credits in the corner: 'Thanks to Jeremy Banks'. I never discovered if he actually was the Jeremy Banks accredited, or whether it was one of his delusions.

I had constant visitors including my mother who came every day on the train, and Trevor who came once or twice a month, when he could get away. My university friend, Rob made a welcome visit. The weeks passed and I still had little grasp of reality. For instance, I believed that ordinary everyday events had a special significance for me. Items of news on the radio for example – Once there was a story about a baby who had been abducted from her home; I believed that I WAS that baby and, when she was found safe and well and returned to her mother, I felt I had 'found myself'. I felt reborn and imbued with a special spiritual elation which lasted for some days.

The pop songs of the time (1971) had particular meaning – "Me and You and a Dog Named Boo" meant to me that Trevor and his friend Dave were travelling down the M1 to visit me. It was not solely my obsession. One young patient was convinced that the song "Tom, Tom, Turn Around" concerned her husband and his supposed infidelity. The husband denied that he had been unfaithful, but Sarah was inconsolable. The television programmes also seemed to be aimed just at me and I believed that all the hospital telephones were bugged. One day I was found on the floor under my bed trying to wrench the air vent from the wall as I thought it was a bugging device.

Finally, the Psychiatrist pressed me to have Electro Convulsive Therapy. As I was under twenty-one, my parents had to give consent and after a lot of anxious consideration they did so. So, ECT became part of my routine.

Always at seven a.m. we were given a cup of tea – except on Tuesdays and Fridays. On those days, all ECT patients were not allowed any food or drink from first thing in the morning. That cup of tea was like a lifeline to me, and oh the pleasurable anticipation of hearing the rattle of the tea trolley getting ever nearer. On Tuesdays and Fridays, the clatter of cups would pass by my room and I'd realize suddenly, with an ice-cold knot in my stomach that it was ECT day. On those days, the poor patients singled out for treatment would not bother to dress, but would queue in hospital dressing- gowns of dull rainbow hues for the initial injections.   How I hated the injections! After an hour or so of agonising waiting, we would be herded unwillingly downstairs to the special ward where long low rubber covered beds, each with a name slotted into the end, awaited us. We would have to lie down on our bed and wait. One by one the beds were wheeled behind curtained partitions and the Asian nurse would roll up our sleeve and tell us to start counting to ten. I never passed the count of three – one, two, three, three …

The first time, I remember waking with such a dark hateful headache that I thought I had died. Then, instantly, with no warning, I was sick all over the floor. Subsequent treatments still caused the headaches, but the sickness passed. Those headaches, they would last all day, like an almighty and never ending sledgehammer battering unceasingly at my brain. The pacing of feet on the corridor was enough to increase the weight of that hammer, and the only acceptable way to bear the day, was sitting passively in a chair awaiting nightfall and the release of sleep.

THE NEST OF SANITY

The ECT treatment however did help rid me of delusions and hallucinations. I no longer believed that Stuart was dead or dying; I no longer felt claustrophobic, or imagined myself flying down hospital corridors. I was, however, shaky and nervous, with constant butterflies in my stomach.

During these weeks I felt a need for religion. I used to go to the hospital chapel and sit quietly breathing in the atmosphere. Also, a fellow patient called Connie would accompany me to the local church, where I felt the service was particularly addressed to me. I did not partake of communion as Connie did, but I felt a closeness and union with God not normally experienced in my healthy state.

Towards the end of July 1971, my sister Caroline, who was training to be a teacher at college in Cheshire, came to stay at my parents' house. She was due to get married on August 7th to a fellow student, to whom she had been engaged for some time. At first it was thought that I would not be well enough to attend the wedding, but as the day approached I was cheered by the news that I could have a day out of the hospital. I assumed Trevor would be there, but was anxious as there was some animosity between him and my future brother-in-law, John.

One sunny day beforehand I remember my sister brought everyone to the hospital grounds and we had a picnic on the grass outside my room. I had never forgiven Caroline for not answering my call for help from Sheffield three months' before and the atmosphere I felt was one of forced joviality and friendliness. My mum however always enjoyed such occasions and it was lovely to see her less strained. The day was spoiled for me when I came out into a bright red sunburn after only a brief spell in the sun – apparently my medication made my skin ultra sensitive to sunlight.

I remember vividly the day my father came to the Clinic to visit me. I had refused to see him while I had been ensconced in my bedroom at home. I hadn't wanted to face up to the effects of his stroke; I was frightened it would be too distressing. The stroke had left his right arm fairly numb; it hung down at a funny angle. He could use it, but had been forced to give up his barber's trade as he was no longer adept with the scissors. My father was quite pessimistic by nature and the stroke left him depressed and disinterested in the future. He refused to cooperate in any rehabilitation programme and passed his days sitting in his fireside armchair watching the new colour television – sport, documentaries and nature programmes, whatever was on at the time. His thoughts were no doubt elsewhere, mainly in his past, thinking of his upbringing in South Wales and his brothers and sisters, now mostly dead.

Dad must have been upset by my refusal to see him and deeply confused and upset by my illness. There had been no history of mental health problems in the family before. I had been the first of his children to reach university and of that he was very proud. I was always very close to my Dad.

That day, I was called downstairs as I had a visitor. I remember skipping down the stairs and stopping, mouth agape, when I saw Dad sitting amongst the potted plants in the reception area. I saw his face light up, and tears sprang to his eyes and mine. I rushed forward for a big hug. There was no need to say much, though we did talk for a while. He cried a little as he left, and we were both overcome at being reunited.

My sister's wedding day came at last, and I nervously bade farewell to the Nurse on duty and left with Trevor to drive home. My legs felt like jelly and I was sure people would notice how ill at ease I was. I had lost weight over the last few months and fitted easily into the long summer dress I had sewn for the ball earlier in the year. (The photos showed me as thin and pale.) It was lovely to see Caroline radiant and happy by John's side. Trevor was very considerate and supportive; otherwise I don't think I could have got through the day. There were not many people attending the ceremony, but I felt extremely anxious and was shocked to see my parents' house seemingly full of strangers. Trevor became a bit disgruntled. (He was a moody and rather unpredictable person. Only months later did I learn that there had been words between Trevor and John and it had been said that Trevor was not welcome at the wedding.) I slipped away from the toasts and went up to my bedroom which I used to share with Caroline. I walked around the room in a daze, fingering ornaments I had collected since childhood and which I was to keep for many years. I felt as though I was in a dream and later was totally relieved to be driving through the hospital gates and back to sanctuary. There, I could retreat back into my shell; no responsibilities, few demands, no decisions to make. I could sleep and forget all that had happened. How safe, secure and protected I felt...

THE NEST OF SANITY

TURN OVER

Slowly, sombrely my eyes see the dim light
The dawning of another day.
Why does my heart fill with fright
Of what lies ahead?
Fear seizes my body
Palpitating my mind.
Quickly, take the tablets
To leave all that behind.
Beating heart quietens
Life's ebb flows
Turn over
To sleep again to hide my sorrows.

Why am I without you?
When with you I am calm.
All my contentment
Vanishes
The moment you leave.
What harm will I come to
Without you?
Turn over
To sleep again to hide my loneliness.

That deep cushioning sleep
Warm, protective, safe.
I could sleep all day.
Turn over
It might all go away.

1971, Churchill Clinic, Harlow

As I gradually got better, I responded more to my surroundings. In Occupational Therapy, I started knitting and took an interest in the various projects of the other patients – rug making, painting, jigsaws. I began to tinker with an old manual typewriter in one of the craft rooms, typing out copies of well-loved poems from a ragged anthology. Then I started writing my own poems, trying to express how I felt and what I had gone through. I loved listening to music and played endless records on an old record player in the lounge. I think some of the patients were irritated with the repetition of the same melodies each day. There was a strange collection of singles and LPs in the Clinic. One which made an impression was 'What are You Doing the Rest of Your Life?' sung by Andy Williams. Another I grew to love was 'New World in the Morning' by Roger Whitaker. Even today this can evoke memories of that time. One of the male nurses, Paul, used to play the piano, trying to encourage a sing song, but the tunes were early seventies music not known to older patients. I occasionally would join in and sing along when feeling in an extrovert mood. This was greeted with clapping and cheers.

The idea arose that there should be general knowledge quizzes. A blackboard and easel was brought into the dining room, with rows of chairs in front. The patients were divided into teams. After a few rounds of questions, it was generally felt that I was a valuable asset to a team: 'We want Rebecca on our side!' The questions asked were amazingly easy for me and I was enjoying myself. The other patients seemed to have an incredible lack of general knowledge, or perhaps their minds were a little clouded due to their medication.

As the weeks passed, I began to take pleasure in the various distractions organised to fill our hours. I was allowed home for brief visits and then for a whole weekend. It seemed very weird to be at home – the reality I knew was *inside* the hospital.

After this first breakdown in 1971, it took me over a year to get completely back to normal. Though in some ways I was never the same again. In hospital, after ECT, you are stripped down to the very soul; bare feelings and emotions are exposed. If you were fond of a fellow patient, you would openly tell them. In group therapy sessions, we were encouraged to reveal our feelings: hatred, despair, anger, revenge, guilt, joy and love. Revealed and exposed to all and sundry you were left vulnerable and unsure. Outside the hospital, I had to build up the barriers necessary for every day social interaction. In a way I still feel that the behaviour inside is more honest – it's a pity we cannot live that way all the time. And what an effort it is to restore those protective barriers and to regain self confidence long since lost.

THE NEST OF SANITY

1971-75: INTERLUDE

I continued taking fairly heavy medication for four years. I felt pretty confident, despite the Psychiatrist's view that my illness was recurrent, that I would not have another breakdown. Surely, I would recognise the signs - weepiness, insomnia, strange thoughts, not coping – and be able to prevent a further relapse into mental illness? I had regular visits to my GP and to Dr. T. during those years. And after a period of building up my confidence again, I did manage to lead a normal active and happy life.

I was allowed to take a year out of University, so I lived with my parents and worked locally as a Council Clerk, doing a typing course in the evenings. When the autumn came in 1972, I resumed my place at Sheffield University, living in a big student house, Florey Lodge. A lot of my old friends had graduated in the meantime and it was quite hard to make new friends as everyone was studying hard as it was their final degree year. The syllabus had altered while I had been sick and I had exam papers specially designated for me. It was a turbulent year in my personal life as Trevor and I had an unsettled relationship, but I managed to complete my course, passed my exams and achieved a BA Dual Honours in Modern History and Politics in the summer of 1973.

For the next two years I trained as a Librarian in Luton and did a Post-Graduate

Diploma in Librarianship at Birmingham Polytechnic. My relations with Trevor continued to be turbulent during that time, but I seemed to cope fairly well. My family and some friends were not very keen on him and I know I lost good friends by sticking with him, but I did feel love for him and no-one could persuade me to leave him, despite his unreliability and crude behaviour. He did try to care for me in his own way. My Dad had been ill and I frequently went down South to visit my family. I maintained a close relationship with Trevor, despite our geographical separation, until early 1975. Then, we finally parted, a break which deeply distressed us both. I felt we had been drifting along in a relationship which had no purpose; neither of us was sure about marriage. I felt I no longer loved him.

For six months, in an effort to forget Trevor, I went out regularly with a Welsh boy called Rhyd. I was studying at college and met him at the local Intervarsity Club. Our social life was busy playing table tennis, dancing at night and watching his favourite cricket and rugby matches. I made new friends through Rhyd and in fact took him to meet my Dad, who was very enthusiastic about our relationship, for he was Welsh himself. I began to feel rather down and cried at any eventuality. Trevor persistently telephoned me, sometimes in tears, as he was so upset about our separation. Finally, I became extremely temperamental and argued irrevocably with Rhyd. It wasn't anything he'd done; I had just used him on the rebound.

THE NEST OF SANITY

That weekend I telephoned and renewed contact with Trevor and started seeing him again. I felt I couldn't help myself. He knew me so well.

I was aware that I was in a confused state, but the GP only gave me more and more pills. I had passed my Post-Graduate exams and now had a temporary bibliographical job at Birmingham University Library, throughout that hot summer (1975). I began to find day to day living difficult to cope with. My nights were restless; I slept little, and when sleep came, my dreams were dramas of confusion, with Trevor's face merging grotesquely with Rhyd's. I felt irritable, shaky and quite ill, with a sore throat and achy limbs. Was it all happening again? What could I do to get out of this mess?

Rebecca Morgan

PART THREE

1975: BIRMINGHAM

The Birmingham streets were crowded with shoppers. Although it was only early September, many people were busily starting their Christmas shopping. I ran my fingers through my unwashed hair and pushed open the glass door into Boots. The pharmacy was downstairs, so I decided to take the escalator. That familiar old cold knot of fear tightened in my stomach sending waves of panic through my body. But my need for those tranquilisers was greater than any fear. I quickly reached into the pocket of my grubby raincoat for my cigarettes.

I stood at the counter and held out my prescription to the girl. She was young and slim but with an acne-d complexion.
"I'm sorry, but you can't smoke in here". She pointed to a large 'No Smoking' sign above the door.
"Well, it's either smoking or screaming, which do you prefer?" I stood my ground.
The girl stared back dumbfounded.
"O.K.", I muttered, and ground the lighted fag end into the white pristine plastic in front of me.
Suddenly, I was aware that everyone was staring – the rows of waiting customers had all turned, some half smiling at the anticipation of a scene.
Unexpectedly, I burst into sobs of tears and was

THE NEST OF SANITY

rescued by Rosemary, a girl I knew slightly, who appeared miraculously from behind the pharmacists' window, and , who, taking me by the arm, led me to a chair at the side of the room. Quickly and without fuss, she pressed a hankie in my hand, saw that my prescription was dispensed with speed and walked me to the door. As I left, I glanced behind, my eyes focussing on the dull brown melted hole in the counter.

****

The buzz of the doorbell interrupted my thoughts. I dragged the arm of the record player across the LP with a grinding scrape and leapt to my feet. The doorbell buzzed again. Wiping the beads of sweat from underneath my fringe, I ran downstairs to the door of the maisonette, and taking a deep breath opened it a fraction. Two gas board officials stood there; the first one with a clip board in his hand. They explained they had come to make safety adjustments to the central heating boiler as arranged. Rather reluctantly I let them into the flat. I was living with a friend while studying at Birmingham Polytechnic for a year.

I left the men removing the vent in the hall and escaped into the lounge. My flatmate was at work and I was on my own that day. I shut the door and leant against it, breathing heavily. So, my time was running out. These men meant business and their business meant my suffering. With some effort I pulled the large leather settee so that it was positioned blocking the opening of the door. I fetched the lightweight kitchen chairs and stacked them on the top of the settee. Hurriedly, I put on a record to hide the noise I was making. I glanced at my watch – blast! It had stopped at 10 a.m. The clock in the little kitchenette off the lounge read 11.15. Hammering noises penetrated the room – the gasmen were trying to get in – if they succeeded, where could I hide? My eyes scoured the room looking for a retreat, but there was none. The hammering grew louder. My breath was coming in gasps and I was dripping with sweat. I scratched the stereo arm across the LP and grabbed the phone.

With trembling hands I rang Trevor's Birmingham office. The ever efficient secretary put me through.
"Hello, Trevor, it's me. You must help me… they're here and they're trying to kill me. Please come, now!!"
"Rebecca, what on earth… calm down? I don't understand who's trying to kill you?"
"Trevor, I can't talk anymore. If they get to me… I'LL HAVE TO KILL MYSELF IF THEY GET NEAR ME… PLEASE COME, PLEASE."
By now I was screaming in fear. I slammed the receiver down. The kitchen clock read 11.25.

By 11.45 a.m. Trevor had arrived – having driven like a maniac across the city. He was let in by the two workmen, who, having finished their task, were on their way out. With great relief, I removed the barriers, let Trevor into the lounge and clung to him, sobbing.

That afternoon, Trevor took me to the Student Health surgery, where I was dispensed some tranquilisers and given a return appointment for a week later. I don't remember much about that visit; I said little and let Trevor do the talking. That night Trevor stayed by my side and finally he fell asleep exhausted. I could not rest; a voice penetrated my thoughts, a repetitive voice intoning names and addresses which I recognised as friends and relatives of mine. The man in the flat downstairs must have stolen my address book and he was even repeating out-of-date addresses which I had previously crossed through. How dare he? I slipped from the bed and regardless of the night time temperatures, hurried downstairs and out of the front door with just a nightie on.

Repeatedly, I pressed the neighbours' doorbell. Finally after a few minutes, Geoff came to the door.
"How dare you steal from me, and nose into my affairs?" I screamed at him.
Though furious at being disturbed, Geoff who had a small baby, tried to keep calm.
"I don't know what you are talking about. Go back to bed, Rebecca, we can talk about it tomorrow."
"NO", I yelled. "How can I sleep when you are going on and on and on...?"
With a start I felt a hand on my shoulder, and with a brief word of apology to Geoff, Trevor led me

away and upstairs to my flat. I cried and protested, but even though Trevor was sympathetic, he did not believe my explanation. No-one believed me: the doctor, Trevor, my friends. I would have to think of a plan; everyone was against me. Perhaps if I turned to my family, they would help. Surely they would help me…

My mother and my eldest brother and his wife drove up to Birmingham two days later after frantic phone calls from Trevor. They managed to persuade me to move lock, stock and barrel home to Hertfordshire. A day or so later after being Sectioned again, I was re-admitted to the Churchill Clinic in Harlow where I had spent four months, four years previously.

THE NEST OF SANITY

1975: HARLOW

Once again I was in a state of delusion. I looked out of the window of my hospital room, seeing the rubble and confusion of a building site as total destruction and devastation. I watched the sun in the sky – it was no longer moving; the earth must be tilted off its axis due to the nuclear war which had just taken place. I was lucky to have survived – more than lucky – in fact, chosen by God to lead the people into a New World. I would be instrumental in recreating this World, for I was God's messenger.

I felt a special closeness to my youngest brother, Graham, who had recently become a Christian. I felt God had a special place for me, and as God's chosen children, Graham and I were kindred spirits. Years later, I tried to feel the fervour which he felt but failed miserably.

I struggled each time the nurses came to inject me. I was being treated with largactyl again and how I fought off those syringes, like a wild animal, biting, scratching and screaming. One time the needle actually broke and the end of it stuck in my bottom. They had to pull it out and it was painful. I swore and shouted out for Stuart or Trevor to come and help me, but no-one came to my aid. No-one listened as I tried to tell them urgently that Jesus wanted ME to save the troubled world.

Rebecca Morgan

POEM

I used to sing songs
Lying on my bed
In the hospital.
I used to walk the floors
At night.
I used to cry and shiver,
Quaver at those needles.
I used to laugh
A laugh of despair.
You never came
Either of you.
I needed you most
But you never came.
"Why?" I asked,
"Never mind" I was told.
I used to cry and shiver
Quaver at those needles.

1975, Churchill Clinic, Harlow

THE NEST OF SANITY

The devastation was immense. Rubble surrounded the only remaining wall, with mud and dust. An old pram was bent in two, fallen by the old green gate. I couldn't believe my old home was gone. I gaped, open-mouthed and horrified. My mother pleaded with me:

"Come on, we'll go in and have a cup of tea." Tea, tea, how could I think of tea, when the big old house was gone, struck by the force of a nuclear bomb?; already Mum's face was wrinkled from the fall-out radiation. I struggled as her arm gently pulled mine, I spat and swore, leaping out of the car and running onto the grass of the lawn, scattered as it was with bricks, splintered wood and glass. Glass, yes, from the windows. I sat with my back to the section of fence which had survived in tact, and stared up at the windows. One side of the house still stood, with windows half smashed and jagged pieces of glass searing across those vacant spaces. From within, ghastly voices, laughing and jeering, and suddenly each vacant window was filled with ugly distorted evil faces all sneering and pointing at me. What a fool I was to think we could survive – maimed and malformed creatures now peopled our earth, our town, my own house. A step on the path at my side; it was Graham, my youngest brother, who was trying to understand the nightmare. Together we knelt; hands clasped and mouthed the Lord's Prayer. A siren wailing, pierced the air. White coated men grasped my arms and steered me to certain death. All I remember of the journey back

to hell is my brother saying over and over again as he clasped my hand,
"It's Graham, I understand. It's Graham, I understand."

Back in the beige-tiled corridors of the Clinic, I understood that my visit home had been disastrous. I was installed back in my small characterless room, where my conversations I knew were bugged. The inmates were plotting my death only a few yards away in the lounge. Quietly, carefully, I crawled under the high bed and tried to pull the bugging device from the skirting board. No, it was no use, it was fixed too firmly. I would have to get some sort of tool, yes a knife from the dining room that was my plan…

The mottled red rash on Dr. T's forehead only reinforced my belief that radiation sickness was beginning. He sat back in his chair.
"So, Rebecca, you believe that you have been sent down to earth to recreate a better world, after the onslaught of some nuclear disaster?"
"Yes, of course, but what's the use? I'm struggling against people who hate me, who daily hurt me and who are plotting to kill me. Leave me alone. Leave me free to put God's will into effect. Please, please."
"OK, don't get upset. Now, we'll give you something to calm you down, so you can have a little sleep. Then, perhaps some tea, eh?"

THE NEST OF SANITY

"No, no, don't!!" I cried, as the nurse held my arm still and the doctor pierced my vein with the inevitable syringe.

HIDDEN TRUTH

I saw that darkness
That total black
Those faces
Leering.
I heard the shots
The bombs
I saw the terror
Of those faces.
I told how I had to cure this,
This mess of a world.
I told how He had chosen
Me.
Now I look back
At that darkness
And realize
One of those faces
Was me.

1975, Churchill Clinic, Harlow

THE NEST OF SANITY

Streaks of light began to pierce the dense blackness which engulfed me. I could feel the perspiration running down my back and dripping off my forehead. It was so hot; the earth's temperature unbalanced by the bomb's effects.
"Wake up love – Rebecca. Here's your mother to see you."
"Hello there, I've brought you some magazines and chocolate. Dad sends his love."
"Go away – I don't want to see you. Can't you leave me alone?"
The nails on my hand tore through her cheek and I was a little surprised to see red as I pulled my hand away.
"Get lost", I shouted, "Leave me alone..."

SOMETIMES

Sometimes
That darkness returns.
It penetrates my mind
And soul.
Endless depths of darkness
Fear and despair.
Alone, alone,
Where are you now?

Sometimes
That feeling takes control.
Oh, to be out of this pain
Which surrounds me.
It penetrates my mind
And soul.
Endless tears and fear
Of life without you.
Alone, alone,
Where are you now?

1975, Churchill Clinic, Harlow

THE NEST OF SANITY

Once more I had to experience the trauma of Electro Convulsive Therapy. This procedure did not get any easier, but in fact did help me by alleviating the delusions and hallucinations from which I was suffering. Gradually, I began to emerge from my psychosis. I became more aware of my surroundings and realised that things had not changed much since my last stay at the Clinic. I recognised many nurses, doctors and even some of the patients.

One character Reginald was in the middle of acrimonious divorce proceedings. His wife wanted a divorce on the grounds of unreasonable behaviour and he was furious. Reginald used to get into violent rages when his wife was mentioned or whenever she crossed his mind. Surprisingly, the rest of the time he seemed a kind and gentle man, who shared with me an interest in and love of the paintings of Vincent van Gogh. I remember a solicitor coming to serve papers on him for the divorce and the poor man went so wild that he had to be physically restrained by two charge nurses. He was soon after injected with a sedating drug.

Meanwhile, I felt empty and inadequate. I had no self confidence and worried about what was going to happen to me. I was cheered up by many visitors. My mum never missed a day, though Trevor never came and my brother Stuart was again abroad. I was really pleased by a surprise visit from my friend from Devon, Steve who travelled up especially. He was feeling unwell most of the time but did seem to be managing. There was a brief letter of sympathy from Rhyd wondering if he could do anything to help, but I sensed he was out of his depth and wanted to cool things.

Sleep still escaped me most nights. I would doze fitfully, finally venturing as far as the nurses' station to sit with the night staff. I could never believe the clock when it read three or four in the morning and for a long time thought that it was fixed at a false time to deceive me. This type of paranoia was common amongst the patients in Churchill. I began to take part in Occupational Therapy projects and began to make a Readicut rug from a kit, to knit and to write more poetry. I had become quite fond of some of the other patients. I even began to write a book in French called "La vie c'est ce qu'on le fait" (Life is what you make it.) I had studied French to A level standard and often had thoughts and dreams in French. On Friday evenings we would have a proper disco with flashing lights (but fortunately no strobes) and modern music. I asked my Mum to bring in my long dresses which were fashionable in the seventies and thus attired I would become quite extrovert and enjoy dancing happily for hours.

Gradually, I was allowed home for visits. I was happy by then to see my Dad who had suffered terribly when I was refusing to see him.

THE NEST OF SANITY

By December 1975 I had become a Day Patient and travelled back and forth from Broxbourne to Harlow three days a week. My brother Stuart was due home for Christmas that year and I was looking forward to seeing him. I also enjoyed seeing my other two brothers, Henry who lived locally and Graham who still lived at home. Stuart was planning to marry in Tasmania in late January and I was determined to attend the wedding if I possibly could. This proved a real incentive to get better. My Mum and I made travelling plans for a three week trip to Australia, my Mum never having been abroad before and never having flown. My Dad sadly was too ill to join us, so the idea was that Graham would keep an eye on Dad while we were gone. The hospital discharged me in time to make the journey and, after some difficulty in getting a visa, all went ahead. I remember how shaky and nervous I felt during my stay over the other side of the world but it was a wonderful experience and a marvellously relaxing holiday for both me and my mother. The wedding was lovely and passed without a hitch and my Sister-in-law's family made us very welcome. My stay there, although I was still on medication, definitely aided my recuperation.

1976-80 INTERLUDE

After our return from Australia, I was uncertain what to do with my life, where to live, what I wanted. Firstly, I spent three months living with my sister Caroline in Manchester. Her and her husband were both teachers, out all day. I found it difficult to get up in the mornings, but eventually I started doing voluntary work in the local Oxfam shop. Also, I resumed driving lessons, which I had given up several months previously. Finally, I came to the decision that I would return to Sheffield, a place where I had found much happiness. I contacted a girlfriend, Jane, who had been a fellow student at Library College in Birmingham and who lived in Sheffield. I began by moving all my belongings to her flat and slept on her floor for two weeks while searching for accommodation.

I had good luck within a week and moved into a bed-sit in Hunters Bar in Sheffield, an area I knew well. The house was shared by several people, most of whom were working. I was shown the ropes by Ralph, a young man of similar age who was very kind to me. I was unemployed for some months and also lacking in confidence, but soon I made friends with new house mates and resumed contact with old friends. I began to go out socially and gradually felt more self assured. Ralph was also out of work and our friendship became companionship and finally love. He was patient, kind and considerate and we had lots in common. How lucky I felt to have found him. His mother had recently suffered a nervous breakdown and I was able to fully understand what she was going through. Late in 1976 I managed to get a job on the Job Creation Scheme, doing advice and information work at a community centre in Broomhall. I was coping with an active life, a demanding job and a happy personal life.

From 1976 to 1980, I did not take any medication at all, and felt fairly well despite major upheavals in my life. I was however very moody and difficult to live with. My father died in 1977, I got married to Ralph in 1978 and I became pregnant in 1979. My father's health had steadily deteriorated since his stroke and his reluctance to take exercise resulted in poor circulation. He was in his late sixties when he was diagnosed with diabetes and had to take tablets; but he consistently refused any form of rehabilitation or activity. Finally his feet and legs became gangrenous, which was painful and upsetting for the whole family. He died, weary and wanting a release from his life of pain, from bronchial pneumonia, in March 1977. He was sixty-eight. He had been a heavy smoker all his adult life. I was obviously very distressed but the family had felt it coming for a long time and therefore felt some relief. My father had wanted to die for a few years and I felt that at last he could have some peace.

Rebecca Morgan

HOSPITAL BEDSIDE

He breathes shallowly.
I watch his face.
Does he even know me now?
He beckons for water.
Gently, I pour a few drops
Into his dribbling mouth.
He nearly chokes,
He cannot breathe,
Hampered by his bronchial chest.

What is he thinking?
He sleeps now.
I keep holding my breath,
Expecting his every one
To be his last.

Is this the man
I loved as a child?
I love more deeply now.
He's lead a troubled life
And always through it,
He's feared the worst.
Why is it he doubted us so much?
Why did he dwell on past misdeeds?

Still, he's peaceful at last.
Perhaps this will be a thankful release
From the pain of his inner world.

Sitting here, alone with him
I secretly hope that

THE NEST OF SANITY

If he has to die soon,
Let him go now,
While I selfishly
Watch his every breath.
I want jealously
To guard over his last few moments
In a way I couldn't do for his first.

1977, Hertford Hospital.

The funeral which took place on a cool rainy March day was attended by all the family, except for Stuart who was unable to return from Australia in time. My life continued in Sheffield. I had a happy and easy going relationship with Ralph, which was a contrast to the ups and downs of my time with Trevor. I was working still in citizen's advice, this time for the Council in Langsett. Ralph and I bought a terraced house in Hunters Bar near our favourite Botanical Gardens, in May 1978 and we quickly settled in, making new friends amongst the neighbours. I was offered a temporary Librarian post at Sheffield University and was pleased to return to my profession. Indeed I became a Chartered Librarian that same year. We had decided we wanted a baby and were happy when I became pregnant two years after getting married. I felt marvellously well and we both looked forward with happy anticipation to the birth of our child.

THE NEST OF SANITY

PART FOUR

1982: FINALE

This takes us back to where I started my story. We have gone full circle covering eleven years of my life. This book was written two years after coming out of Middlewood Hospital, and I felt well, confident and capable. Steven was two years old, a bright and lively little boy who seemed not to have suffered too much from my abandonment in the early days of his life. I was taking a minimum dosage of drugs and it had been recommended that I take those indefinitely. Deep down in my subconscious there was an ever present fear of some sort of recurrence of mental illness. In some ways, I felt that it was inevitable that I would fall from the nest of sanity once more. But I hoped that this time I would stay secure from madness for the rest of my life. As a doctor once said to me, if I did become ill again, at least I had the consolation that I have always got better. That gave me the hope to carry on...

2007: EPILOGUE

Twenty-Five years have passed since I wrote this story. On the whole I kept very well during this time, but was always a worrier and I still sometimes got very anxious.
But yes, I did fall from the nest once again, but this was due to very stressful circumstances which I will tell you about.

A year after Steven's birth, the Mother and Baby Unit I had been in, closed down and mothers had to be transferred to Rotherham to get that type of care. There was a lack of groups supporting such mothers so from 1981-87 I set up and ran a Post-Natal Depression Support Group in Sheffield with a good friend Agnes Burns. We had both experienced PND and were able to share our experiences with other Mums, helping them to cope. We regularly gave support to Mums, were interviewed on local radio and once did a talk to 450 midwives in Cardiff about our experiences. Helping others in this way helped me too. Meanwhile I was practising yoga and keep fit to try and relax. I was feeling a lot better and very rarely felt depressed. However this didn't mean I wasn't anxious or nervous about things which happened in my life during this time. Steven was growing up and was quite a sensitive child, though very bright and thoughtful. In 1987 I finally secured a part-time job as a Librarian for Sheffield City Council. This was the start of a new career lasting over 20 years.

THE NEST OF SANITY

As I previously mentioned we decided not to have more children as the risk of PND or a breakdown of some sort was too great. (In fact the odds were an 85% chance of a Psychotic episode happening again.) Ralph was made redundant in 1982 and together we set up our own business which continues to this day. These were busy times during which I campaigned for CND, joined a writing group and a women's group. Ralph's elderly parents were brought up from Hampshire to live near us in Sheffield, though sadly Ralph's Dad died three years later. Over the years we saw a lot of our families and spent many happy summers with my mother. Mum found a new freedom after my Dad died, and travelled regularly around the country happily visiting her children and 10 grandchildren. I also found the experience of motherhood brought me closer to my sister and we began to keep in regular contact.

In 1995-6 Steven began experiencing periods of depression, which culminated in a breakdown in May 1998 (when he was eighteen) and eventually a diagnosis of Bipolar Disorder (Manic Depression). This was one of the hardest things I had ever coped with. I would rather I had been ill myself than my own son, and felt guilty that I had either passed on my illness to him genetically or affected him by the way I had brought him up.

Rebecca Morgan

TEENAGE BREAKDOWN

From blue-eyed babe
Cheerful tot
To clever young boy.
Too sensitive those eyes
Those feelings hurt.
So adolescent angst
Comes true.

Weary face, pale and thin
Body lays and trembles
Mouth dry, chemicals race
Stomach rises to anxiety.

He cries
Huddles on the floor
Can I bear this?

With anguish I search my guilt –
Where lies the fault?
Was I too caring?
Was I too harsh?
Have I revealed
My years of stress
Too openly?

He's been "lonely forever"
And "unhappy for years".

I long to hug
And care those fears away

THE NEST OF SANITY

But I am powerless.
I can do nothing
But listen and watch...
And wait for time to heal.

May 1998, Burbage Ward, Michael Carlisle
Centre, Sheffield

This worry culminated in me having another breakdown that May (1998) and spending six days in Whiteley Wood Psychiatric Clinic in Sheffield. This was set in lovely grounds, but was a nightmare of a place. My behaviour had become peculiar and I threatened to commit suicide, asking my husband to hide all my tablets so I would not be able to reach them. I took to Steven's bed (he was in hospital) but I could not sleep and was not rational, at one point angrily telling my best friend to "p*** off" when she telephoned for the ambulance to get me admitted. My husband, Ralph was distraught, as for a few days both his son and his wife were on Psychiatric wards.

In the Clinic things were very confusing. It was hard to tell who were staff and who were patients. There were some very disturbed patients and I was twice threatened with a knife. I started smoking and as a result, when the public phone booth was set alight, I was accused of arson. I had belongings stolen including personal items. I was again paranoiac, thinking there was a plot against me. Many friends came to visit but often I would just swear at them in disgust, something I normally would not do. I tried to keep it a secret from my mother, who was beginning to be confused at the start of her dementia, and I was very upset when a mutual friend told Mum what had happened. I felt Mum was not up to coping with the fact that both Steven and I had cracked up. I became quite hysterical and had to be

THE NEST OF SANITY

subdued. I had the feeling of panic in my stomach constantly. I was sometimes unable to pass water, and had dreadful insomnia. My mind was racing and I started writing my second book. This book was to describe my hell at seeing Steven on a Psychiatric Ward, and the struggle he was going through to come to terms with his illness. It didn't help the situation that I was taken off all my medication at the Clinic. After only a few days however I was discharged back to my home, with Steven still an in-patient at another Clinic. My husband Ralph was marvellous and cared for me as best he could with great help and support from friends and neighbours. In return, I was impatient with Ralph and belittled him at every opportunity.

Thus, I had fallen from the nest of sanity again; despite thinking I could have prevented such an occurrence. Luckily for me and the family I was able to avoid the extremes of the illness by taking extra doses of Stelazine (Trifluoperazine) a medicine used for the treatment of Schizophrenia which had helped me so much since my postnatal breakdown. However, I had no self-confidence and I was very shaky and weak. My son's recovery was gradual and so was mine, but eventually with some time off work we were both progressing. Then in 1999, just before his nineteenth birthday, when Steven was applying for a place at University, he was involved in a serious road traffic accident. He nearly died that night and was in intensive care for a while with a severe head injury. I have never forgotten that awful experience. This second blow in two years had a strong effect on my nerves, but Steven made an excellent recovery and moved on to make great academic and social achievements of which we are very proud.

THE NEST OF SANITY

INTENSIVE CARE

A fear so deep I've never known
Came upon me on that day
You nearly left
You nearly died
Life had all but ebbed away.

But, fighter to the core
You rallied round
You reached for life
And searched for love profound –

We have that love
We give that love
And I know it is returned.

My darling son,
My precious boy
You bear your pain with courage
Which gives me special pride.
You chose to stay
You chose to live –
Take shelter by my side.

January 1999 Hallamshire Hospital, Sheffield

Rebecca Morgan

Now in 2007, I have held down a successful professional post for 20 years and most of the time I cope very well. I have a very busy life, taking a carefully balanced prescription of tablets. I generally feel content and although I have days when things do not go well, and I feel under pressure or stress, in no way do I experience the type of depression of my past. The chemical imbalance in my brain, if that is what it is, is remedied by my medication and I thank Dr. Sneddon for prescribing it all those years ago. I have come to terms with taking medication and it does not bother me at all. In a time when stigma is still attached to mental illness, I have never minded talking about my experiences and I regard my four breakdowns as equivalent to having four broken limbs. I used to hate myself when I was younger, now I like myself much better.

The life in a Psychiatric hospital soon becomes a safe environment. As a patient one becomes used to the routines and every day activities. You are to a certain extent institutionalised and you become frightened to leave that security. In order to mix again in the outside world you have to rebuild layers of social awareness, and that is difficult.

I feel more should be done to increase people's knowledge and understanding of mental illness in all its forms for after all, such illness is increasingly common amongst both men and women. One positive result of having been through and recovered from four breakdowns is that I feel I know myself very well. I have managed to moderate my personality a fraction but basically it is hard to change oneself. Sometimes I get rather hyperactive and sometimes I am low, but I deal with this in several ways. I get as much sleep as I can (the tablets cause drowsiness), though still sometimes suffering periods of insomnia. I exercise with keep fit and regular swimming. I try to eat healthily and write a diary and a journal regularly. And above all, I share my problems with family and close friends without whom I would not manage to keep going. I feel I have come to terms with my depression and although still 'a worrier' I do manage to cope with every day stress much better than I ever used to. In a world where mental illness is still regarded with hostility, prejudice, ignorance and shame I feel it is important to talk about it and write about it openly, honestly and without embarrassment.

Through my breakdowns I have suffered much unhappiness and emotional suffering but this means that I do value real happiness and take pleasure in small things. I have matured into a person with more self confidence, although sometimes it does desert me! In many situations this type of illness is worse for close family and friends, who are bewildered and see things that are very disturbing and upsetting. Each time I was ill, my family especially suffered pain while I was in my own weird world. I have become closer to my brothers and my sister in recent years and they are a wonderful support to me.

I intend that my story will be a positive one – yes, you can get better from a Psychiatric breakdown and lead a fulfilling and normal life; yes you can learn to cope with a mental health problem or condition with good support from family and friends. The first step towards getting better is to admit there is a problem. Remind yourself that worrying is a complete waste, a destructive thing which has no effect on the object of all the worry. Try to write about your problems; this is a cathartic and satisfying experience. Avoid the danger of bottling up your anxieties which cumulatively can result in mental breakdown. Talking to someone about it means sharing your experience with others which enables one to get one's own life in proportion. I don't know all the answers and sometimes these things can be very complex, but I hope my story will give you hope.

Finally I can say that I have managed to cope this year with the death of my lovely Mum after her long struggle with Alzheimer's disease. It has been hard but I welcome her release from the pain of that fearful disease; it's to her and my Dad that I dedicate this book.

****

THE NEST OF SANITY

APPENDIX 1: DOCTORS' LETTERS

Extract from a letter to Rebecca from Dr. H. J. Tollinton, Consultant Psychiatrist, dated 3rd March 1982:
"I don't think we ever reached an entirely satisfactory classification for the kind of illness that you had. As you will probably remember, it was not exactly the same in its features in the two episodes in 1971 and 1975. The first illness we finally described as Schizophreniform, query secondary to drug ingestion, and the second as Reactive Excitation/Psychogenic Psychosis. The first illness was marked by auditory and possibly visual hallucinations and confusion of your thinking, as well as a strange feeling that everyday events were of special significance for you. In 1975, you seemed to be much more disturbed by your illness and your behaviour seemed much more difficult to explain. However, once more you were hallucinating, but your thoughts were perhaps less confused. On both occasions you were treated with Electro Convulsive Therapy and major tranquilisers, together with some anti depressants.

I think that most people nowadays would probably include both these illnesses as probably of a Schizophrenic kind, and if not, perhaps describe them as an unsatisfactory compromise – Schizoaffective. I am afraid that this is an area where there is much uncertainty in Psychiatry. Princess Alexandra Hospital, Harlow, 1982.

APPENDIX 1 continued

Extract from a letter to Rebecca from Dr. Joan Sneddon, Senior Lecturer in Psychiatry, University of Sheffield, dated 27th April, 1982.

"I looked after Rebecca during her last Psychiatric illness which was associated with the birth of her baby. She was perfectly well during the pregnancy. Her symptoms started two days after the birth and she was admitted to hospital eight days later.
Rebecca had a serious Psychiatric illness and was an in-patient for three months; her treatment with drugs and ECT was very successful. I saw her regularly after discharge from the ward, as illness associated with childbirth often has relapses before full recovery occurs. She is now well.

This seemed a typical Puerperal Psychosis, but she has had two previous attacks of Psychiatric illness not associated with childbirth, treated in another city. So, it seems likely that childbirth, with its rapid hormonal changes triggered off another attack.

I look forward to reading her book and would like this opportunity to tell readers that acute Psychiatric illness associated with childbirth, however severe, has an excellent recovery rate."

Middlewood Hospital, Sheffield, 1982.

THE NEST OF SANITY

APPENDIX 1 continued

Letter from Rebecca's GP Dr. G. Linnard
Sheffield, dated 26/11/07

"I have known Rebecca since 1997 when I moved
to Sheffield and she became my patient. Despite
the long documented history of mental illness
classified as Hebephrenic Schizophrenia*,
Rebecca has remained well the majority of the
time I have known her. Her last episode of
Psychotic illness occurred in 1998 and was
triggered when her son had a breakdown. At that
time, Carol was extremely agitated with marked
pressure of speech and difficulty in sleeping. She
did require admission to a Psychiatric hospital to
stabilise her condition.

Since then Rebecca has remained extremely well.
She continues to work and run the family home.
One of the most important factors that have
enabled her to remain so well is her readiness to
accept her diagnosis. She understands the need
for her medication and by taking it regularly has
stayed mentally well and stable for nearly 10
years."

*Hebephrenic Schizophrenia means intermittent
and recurring episodes of a Schizophrenic type.

APPENDIX 2: POEMS OF PSYCHOSIS

By sharing the following poems written during periods of Psychosis, I hope to add another dimension to this rational account of my illness. They may be largely nonsense but it reflects my weird thinking when Psychotic.

TO STUART: LOVE IS DEAD

Hope springs forth
But love is dead.
Life is only
In another's head.

Why doest follow?
Lead me home
Help me from
This earthly moan.

My love has gone
And pride despairs.
My love has gone
Where are my tears?

A love so true
And yet so wild
A love so true
Another's child.

Churchill Clinic, Harlow   1971

THE NEST OF SANITY

FOR MY BROTHER STUART

Sonic stillness long resounds
Air which freshly falls as dew.
Water feels the earthly gaze
Of sun, the yellow and the blue.

Pianissimo sounds true
The dark and sombre hue
Of life amongst the few,
Of life amongst the few.

Can gladness toll from bells above?
Or is it only earthly love
Which bridges feelings softly told
And fellowship of love of old.

The ones I pray to see are those
Who are so dear to me.
The fellow sufferers of this world
Require God's aid to make them free.

Churchill Clinic, Harlow   14/10/75

Rebecca Morgan

TO REGINALD: DEFINITION OF LOVE (van Gogh)

Sunflowers be they not,
Sunflowers be they soon,
But life is not all death.
And love comes from a womb.

I feel the light that dies,
I know the mind which falls,
But heaven helps the fallen ones
And others whom He galls.

Churchill Clinic, Harlow   10/11/75

THE NEST OF SANITY

FOR STEVE

The vicious handshake wearily dies
And all the light is filled
With joys:
Joys which feeling can't erase,
Nor believing feelings done.

The world is true:
But life goes on, and music,
Like the sirens wail.
I feel the way,
I feel the way,
But is it all too soon?

The mind is mindful,
Love is great,
But fear is like
Your handshake.

Don't miss me more
Don't miss me less
My feelings can't erase.

Churchill Clinic, Harlow, 10/11/75

Rebecca Morgan

TO REGINALD, ON WAKING

Yawns subside
But you shall glide

None is all;
All is rest;
Rest is full;
Brain is dead.
Life is love
And love –
Is dread.

I know I am smiling,
Perhaps I am crying.
But I know why it's BOTH;
I'm frightened of dying
In the oven I'm frying.

I know:
I am SAFE.

Churchill Clinic, Harlow, 11/11/75

THE NEST OF SANITY

TO MY SISTER CAROLINE, with photo by John

I love your eyes,
And freckles too –
I wish I knew you –
Really you.

I know I'm lost
But in no pain.
Let's forget the past
And start again.

You barefoot girl
I feel you're mine
And knowing comes
Of light divine.

That light divine
Can be yours too
Are you a Christian
Martyr true?

Need I say more?
I've lost the rhyme
I'll finish this
Another time.

Churchill Clinic, Harlow   11/11/75

Rebecca Morgan

TO TREVOR: A Song of Love and Hate (as per L.
Cohen)

I'm as normal as I can be,
I'm as normal as a tree.
I'm as normal as a butterfly,
Who else is there but me?

You're as normal as you can be,
You're normal as my tree.
You're as normal as a scatterbrain
Who spills his cup of tea.

(I love you and
I love the trees.
And I love the butterfly
Do you love me?)

Churchill Clinic, Harlow 11/11/75

THE NEST OF SANITY

TO ROB

I know you now,
I never did –
I felt your world
Would really rid
Me of my own.
I hope that life
Is good for you
So come and see
Me very soon.
But home is best,
And there I'll be
As soon as I
Can plainly see –
THE TRUTH.

Churchill Clinic 11/11/75

TO STUART

I know to give is not to take
I know to love is not to make
But when I fearful hear your tread
The bus jolts on and I am dead.

Dead for you, with all my heart.
Christ is blue, the yawning starts.
The party felt like never more,
But you are coming, you are sure.

Churchill Clinic, Harlow   12/11/75   7a.m.

THE NEST OF SANITY

TO JEREMY

The sight of you
Can make me feel
The way I am:
And that is REAL.

The sight of you
Can make me sleep.
The land of dreams
Is yours to keep.

Churchill Clinic, Harlow   12/11/75

TO RHYD

Typing chores are feeling fine
This is love, oh so sublime.
This is love
And don't you know?
The doctor's on go slow.

Go slow, go fast.
Oh, will it last?
Go up, go down
Oh, will I frown?

The need to read
Is so divine.
That light obscure
May blot this line.

Churchill Clinic, Harlow 12/11/75

THE NEST OF SANITY

TO REGINALD

I'm not fully awake,
To Reginald I'll send a cake;
A cake for his birthday tea;
 And then he can sit by the sea.

January wind blows cold
In England as of old.
I feel the way you are
And now I feel the STAR –
(As in the Bible)

The star to guide your hand,
A law of God's command.
The hand is just at seven –
And we'll all go to heaven.

(But NOT as the Jehovah Witnesses preach it.)

Churchill Clinic, Harlow 14/11/75

FOR JEREMY

Time passes,
Time passes
Laughs and glasses
Of wine.

Life passes,
Life passes
Sometimes lassies
Out of time.

Love passes,
Love passes
Will you ever more
Be mine?

Hope passes,
Hope passes
What could I do
Without time?

Churchill Clinic, Harlow   18/11/75

THE NEST OF SANITY

TO TREVOR

To you a key
To me a tree
A tree of death
A tree of life

To you a flower
To me a rose
A rose in bloom
A rose that wilts

To you a lorry
To me a car
Oh, what and why
Can we see so far?

Churchill Clinic, Harlow 20/11/75

THE NEST OF SANITY

TO TREVOR

Without you, I am nothing:
An empty fallen shell
Which blasts blearily
Into this world of hell.

With you I am <u>someone,</u>
Small, hopefully kind
Who knows she has
A darling, and needs not one to find.

Churchill Clinic, Harlow   26/11/75

FEAR

Why do these fears assail me?
Never quieten my mind.
Fear of failure, guilt and pain
Cuts me like a knife.

I know not
Whence I came
I know not
Where I go
But here is life
And ever present
 Fear.

Doubts creep and crawl
In the pit of my stomach.
Shyness, words do not easily come.
Crying, fear even of the sun.

Why do I suffer so?
When life is essentially good.
Be gone fears and trust in God.

Middlewood Hospital, 19/03/80

THE NEST OF SANITY

APPENDIX 3:   USEFUL ORGANISATIONS

RETHINK
 0845 456 0455
www.rethink.org.uk

DEPRESSION ALLIANCE
0845 123 2320
www.depressionalliance.org.uk

MEET A MUM (MAMA)
0845 120 3746
www.mama.co.uk

MANIC DEPRESSION FELLOWSHIP
0845 634 0540
www.mdf.org.uk

MIND
0845 766 0163
www.mind.org.uk

SANE
0845 767 8000
www.sane.org.uk

SAMARITANS
0845 790 9090
www.samaritans.org

www.ingramcontent.com/pod-product-compliance
Lightning Source LLC
Chambersburg PA
CBHW022157080426
42734CB00006B/471